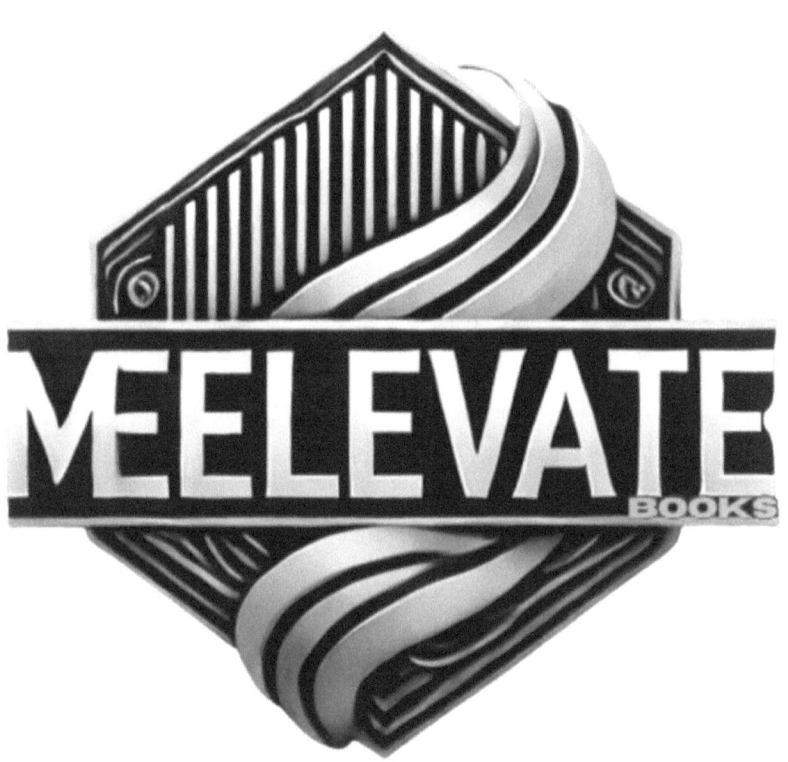

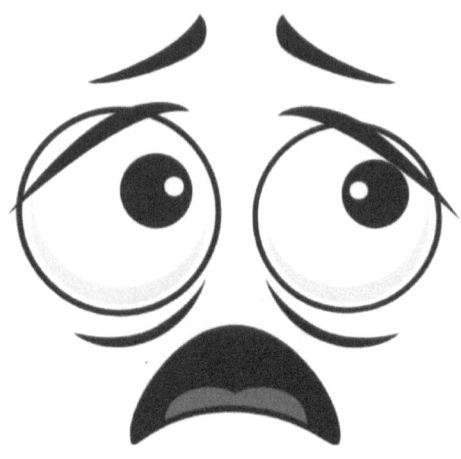

UNLOCKING SERENITY: A GUIDE TO LETTING GO OF WORRY

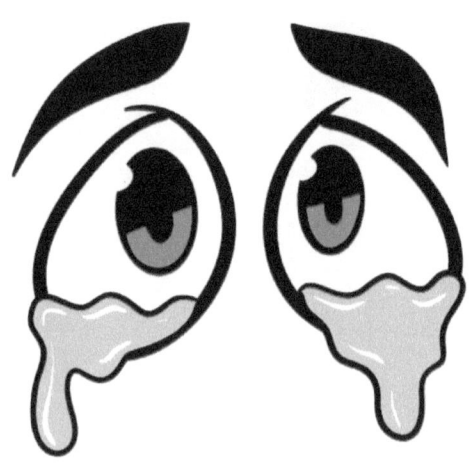

Unlocking Serenity: A Guide to Letting Go of Worry"

RICKEY DAVIS JR

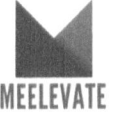

COPYRIGHT

Copyright © 2023 by MEELEVATE LLC. All rights reserved.

No part of this book may be reproduced, stored in a retrieval system, or transmitted in any form or by any means—electronic, mechanical, photocopying, recording, or otherwise—without prior written permission from the publisher, except for brief quotations in reviews or articles.

First Edition: 2023 – UPDATE 2025
Published by MEELEVATE LLC

The author has made every effort to ensure the accuracy of the information contained in this book. However, this book is provided "as is," without any warranties, express or implied. The author and publisher assume no responsibility for errors, omissions, or outcomes resulting from the use of the information provided.

ISBN: 979-8374243642
Imprint: Independently Published

DEDICATION

This book is dedicated to those who have struggled with worry but continue to push forward despite their fears. To the seekers of peace, the dreamers longing for serenity, and the warriors of personal growth—you are not alone.

To my children, who remind me every day of the importance of perseverance and love, and to everyone who has ever felt weighed down by doubt, may this book serve as a guide to unlocking the calm and clarity within you.

And to *MEELEVATE BOOKS*, a movement built on:

M - Mindfulness: Staying present in the journey of personal growth.
E - Endurance: Building resilience to overcome obstacles.
E - Empowerment: Gaining the confidence to take charge of your life.
L - Learning: Embracing growth through knowledge and experience.
E - Emotional Resilience: Adapting and thriving despite hardships.
V - Vision: Setting a clear purpose and goals for your journey.
A - Authenticity: Living true to your values and beliefs.
T - Transformation: Striving for meaningful change.
E - Empathy: Cultivating understanding and compassion.

To all who read this, I hope this book helps you find the peace, strength, and clarity you deserve.

— **Rickey Davis Jr.**

TABLE OF CONTENTS

- Copyright
- Dedication
- Table of Contents
- Introduction:
- Understanding Worry
- Chapter 1: Recognizing Worry
- Chapter 2: Science of Worry and Stress
- Chapter 3: Mindfulness vs. Worry
- Chapter 4: Self-Compassion
- Chapter 5: Reframing Thoughts
- Chapter 6: Managing Worry
- Chapter 7: Emotions in Worry
- Chapter 8: Building Resilience
- Chapter 9: Inner Peace and Serenity
- Chapter 10: Maintaining a Worry-Free Mindset
- Techniques for Reducing Worry
- BONUS

INTRODUCTION

Unlocking Serenity: A Guide to Letting Go of Worry by Rickey Davis Jr and MEELEVATE BOOKS. is a personal development book designed to help readers break free from the cycle of worry and reclaim control over their thoughts, emotions, and overall well-being. Worry can negatively impact every aspect of life—relationships, health, and personal growth—but with the right mindset and strategies, it can be managed effectively.

This book presents a comprehensive **20-step plan** to guide readers through understanding and overcoming worry. It explores key areas such as:

- Recognizing the signs of worry and its impact
- Practicing mindfulness to stay present and grounded
- Developing self-compassion to foster inner peace
- Reframing negative thoughts to create a more positive outlook
- Implementing practical strategies to manage daily stressors

Beyond managing worry, this book emphasizes **self-care, resilience, and emotional balance**. Readers will learn how to navigate difficult situations, cultivate mindfulness, and maintain a **worry-free mindset** as lifelong practice.

Written in a clear and accessible style, *Unlocking Serenity* provides **practical examples, exercises, and actionable tips** to help readers take control of their mental and emotional well-being. The ultimate goal of this book is to **empower you**—to shift from a place of worry to a state of **calm, confidence, and serenity**.

UNDERSTANDING THE CYCLE OF WORRY

Worry can take a serious toll on both mental and physical health. Research shows that chronic worrying contributes to conditions such as **high blood pressure, heart disease, and diabetes**, while also increasing the risk of **anxiety and depression**.

On a mental level, excessive worry can make it difficult to **focus, stay present, and complete daily tasks**, often leading to feelings of **overwhelm and stress**. Emotionally, it can result in **exhaustion, hopelessness, and a sense of being trapped** in negative thought patterns.

Physically, worry often manifests through symptoms like **headaches, muscle tension, fatigue, and even digestive issues**. Over time, these symptoms can weaken the body and exacerbate underlying health conditions.

Spiritually, chronic worry can create feelings of **disconnection, doubt, guilt, or shame**, making it harder to trust in a higher power or personal faith. It can also disrupt inner peace, leaving individuals feeling **lost or uncertain** in their journey.

From a **confident perspective**, excessive worry can lead to **self-doubt and indecisiveness**, making it difficult to trust one's instincts. It often fuels **worse-case scenario thinking**, where the mind fixates on **imagined disasters** rather than realistic outcomes, increasing feelings of fear and anxiety.

The impact of worry is far-reaching, affecting the **mind, body, and spirit**. That's why it is crucial to develop **healthy coping strategies**—whether through **mindfulness, movement, reframing negative thoughts, or seeking professional support**. By understanding the cycle of worry, you can begin to break free from its grip and reclaim control over your well-being.

A PERSONAL STORY ON WORRY

Worry is something that has run through my family for as long as I can remember. I've witnessed it in my grandparents, my mother, and even among friends and extended family. I've seen it play out in classrooms as a student, where the fear of failure would weigh on us even when we tried to focus.

For me, worry has been a constant companion throughout my life. As a single, full-time dad, I've faced my share of struggles—worrying if I'm good enough, wondering if I'm a good father, and questioning whether I'm providing enough for my kids. I've worried about being behind on child support, my bills, my relationships, and not having a stable income or a partner by my side.

Worry has often led me into a cycle of **insecurities** and **depression**, but it wasn't until I started reflecting on these emotions that I realized just how harmful this constant anxiety is. It's a common experience for many people today. We worry about our jobs, our income, and how we will provide for our families.

I know I'm not alone in this. Worry is universal, but its weight varies from person to person. I've learned that it's not just a personal issue—it's a **generational one**. Worrying is something that's often passed down, and breaking that cycle can seem impossible. But I've also learned that **worry doesn't solve problems**. In fact, it only brings **negative energy** and keeps you trapped in a cycle of fear.

Through my personal experience, research, and even the teachings in the Bible, I've come to understand that worry isn't the answer. It's a challenge, no doubt, especially when it's ingrained in us for generations. But I've realized that when I allow myself to worry, I'm choosing to operate on a **negative frequency**—and it doesn't get me anywhere.

This is why I wrote this book. I know that there are many people out there, like me, who have struggled with worry and feel like it's a part of their DNA. Whether it's affecting you personally or has been a burden on your family for generations, I believe there's a way to break the cycle.

Sometimes, we also find ourselves worrying about our loved ones who have passed away. For years, we can linger in that pain and find it hard to let go. Losing someone we care about is one of the hardest things to accept, and often, the weight of grief turns into worry about what might have been.

Additionally, we worry about family members who might be struggling with addiction, caught in the streets, or incarcerated. These worries can feel endless as we wonder about their safety, well-being, and future. But in some cases, even the people we worry about—like those battling addiction or who are incarcerated—are experiencing worry of their own.

As single parents or as a family unit, we often find ourselves worrying about whether our significant other is being faithful, or if the friends we have are truly trustworthy. We worry about how others perceive us, what they think, or what they say behind our backs. The list of worries is long, and it's deeper than we realize.

That's why I believe this topic is so important—it's something we need to talk about more openly. I also think we need to start addressing worry from an early age. If we can teach children in elementary school all the way through high school and college about how to evaluate obstacles instead of worrying about them, they will grow up to be better equipped adults. They'll learn to evaluate situations with clarity, not fear, and in turn, pass this wisdom down to the next generation.

CHAPTER 1: RECOGNIZING THE SIGNS OF WORRY

RECOGNIZING THE SIGNS OF WORRY

Worry is a natural human response, and it can affect various aspects of our lives, from daily tasks to relationships, friendships, work, and even our environment. However, it's important to understand that concern can motivate us to act. Worry often creates more problems than solutions. It can impact on our emotional and mental health in ways that we may not immediately recognize, making it essential to identify and address it early.

As human beings, it's okay to feel concerned or anxious about certain situations. This is part of our survival instinct and drives us to act. But the challenge lies in distinguishing between healthy concern and excessive worry. Worrying excessively about things we cannot control can lead to long-term emotional, physical, and mental consequences.

Recognizing the signs of worry is the first step in addressing it before it spirals into more significant mental health concerns. Some common signs that worry is becoming overwhelming include:

- **Constant, excessive worrying or rumination**: When worry consumes your thoughts and leads to repetitive, unproductive thinking. You might find yourself replaying the same scenarios or worrying about things that are unlikely to happen.

- **Difficulty concentrating or staying focused**: Worry can create a mental fog, making it hard to focus on tasks at hand, whether it's at work, school, or in personal interactions. This distraction can hinder your ability to be productive and engaged.

- **Irritability or mood swings**: Chronic worrying can lead to emotional exhaustion, causing you to feel irritable, anxious, or moody. The weight of your thoughts can make even small situations feel overwhelming.

- **Physical symptoms**: Worry doesn't just affect the mind—it manifests physically, too. Muscle tension, headaches, fatigue, and even digestive issues are common physical symptoms linked to prolonged worry. These symptoms are often the body's response to the stress that accompanies excessive thinking.

- **Insomnia or difficulty sleeping**: When worry runs rampant, it can keep you up at night, preventing restful sleep. The inability to shut off your thoughts can lead to restlessness, and over time, a lack of sleep can exacerbate feelings of anxiety and stress.

By recognizing these signs, individuals can take proactive steps to manage their worry before it escalates. Early intervention is key, and there are several strategies to consider:

- **Practice stress management techniques**: Regular mindfulness practices, like deep breathing or meditation, can help calm the mind. Additionally, finding time for relaxation and physical exercise can alleviate physical symptoms, such as muscle tension, and improve overall well-being.

- **Seeking professional support**: If worry interferes with your ability to function, it may be time to consult with a professional. Therapy, such as cognitive-behavioral therapy (CBT), can help individuals reframe negative thought patterns, while counseling can provide a safe space to express emotions and find coping strategies.

- **Lifestyle changes**: Small adjustments to daily habits can make a significant difference. Creating a structured routine, setting boundaries, prioritizing self-care, and getting enough sleep can all contribute to reducing overall stress and minimizing worry.

In addition to recognizing your own signs of worry, it's equally important to recognize these signs in others. If you notice someone in your life displaying these behaviors, it can be helpful to approach them with empathy and support. Sometimes, just talking to someone about their worries can be the first step toward healing. Encouraging them to seek professional help, practice relaxation techniques, or adopt healthier coping strategies can make a world of difference.

The key takeaway is that worry doesn't have to control our lives. By identifying the signs early and addressing them in healthy ways, we can prevent worry from becoming an overwhelming force. Whether through personal strategies or professional support, managing worry is essential to maintaining mental, physical, and emotional well-being. Taking the first step toward recognizing and addressing worry can ultimately lead to a more peaceful, centered life.

10-STEP ACTIVITY PLAN TO MANAGE WORRY

1. **Identify Your Worries**
   Start by writing down the specific things you are worried about. Reflect on both immediate and long-term concerns. This simple act of journaling helps you externalize your thoughts and see them more clearly, making it easier to analyze which worries are valid and which ones may be exaggerated or unfounded.
2. **Differentiate Between Concern and Worry**
   Ask yourself if your worry is leading to productive action or if it's just consuming your mind. Write down whether your thoughts are problem-solving (concern) or rumination (worry). Recognizing the difference helps you focus on addressing what you can control.
3. **Challenge Negative Thoughts**
   When you catch yourself spiraling into worry, pausing and challenging your thoughts. Ask: "Is this worry realistic? What's the evidence for and against this worry?" Try to reframe negative thoughts by looking for alternative, more balanced perspectives.
4. **Practice Deep Breathing or Meditation**
   Engage in deep breathing exercises or mindfulness meditation for at least 5–10 minutes. These techniques help calm your mind and reduce the physical effects of worry, such as muscle tension and anxiety. Use guided meditation apps or simple breathing techniques (e.g., inhale for 4 counts, hold for 4 counts, exhale for 4 counts) to anchor yourself in the present moment.
5. **Engage in Physical Activity**
   Exercise is a powerful tool for reducing worry and stress. Go for a walk, take a yoga class, or engage in any physical activity you enjoy. Exercise releases endorphins, which help elevate mood and reduce anxiety, while also helping you gain a sense of control over your body and mind.

6. **Create an Action Plan for Worries You Can Control**
   For the worries that are within your control (e.g., work tasks, finances, health), break them down into manageable steps. Write a specific action plan to tackle each one, outlining what you need to do, when you will do it, and any resources you may need. Taking actionable steps gives you a sense of empowerment and reduces the power of worry.
7. **Set Boundaries for Worry Time**
   Allocate a specific "worry time" for yourself. Set aside 15–20 minutes in the day to reflect on your worries. Outside of this designated time, gently redirect your thoughts to something else, practicing mindfulness and letting go of concerns during non-worry time. This practice allows you to limit the impact worry has on your day.
8. **Reach Out for Support**
   Talk to a trusted friend, family member, or counselor about your worries. Sometimes, sharing your concerns with someone else can provide a new perspective and reduce the emotional weight you carry. Whether you need advice or simply a listening ear, social support can act as a powerful tool to combat worry.
9. **Practice Gratitude**
   Start or end your day by writing down three things you're grateful for. Gratitude helps shift focus from what's causing worry to what's going well in your life. This shift in perspective can help you feel more balanced and reduce the intensity of negative thoughts.
10. **Developing a Self-Care Routine**
    Make self-care a non-negotiable part of your routine. This could include activities such as reading, taking a warm bath, spending time with loved ones, or engaging in a hobby. Self-care nurtures your emotional and physical well-being, providing you with the resilience to manage worry over time.

How to Use This Plan

- **Daily Practice**: Commit to practicing one or more of these steps every day to reduce the frequency and intensity of your worries.
- **Weekly Reflection**: At the end of each week, reflect on your progress. Which techniques worked best? Where can you improve?
- **Consistency is Key**: The more consistent you are with these practices, the more you'll begin to notice a positive shift in your mindset.

By incorporating these activities into your routine, you can take control of your worries, reduce their impact on your life, and foster a more peaceful and balanced mindset.

CHAPTER 2: THE SCIENCE OF WORRY AND STRESS

Worry and stress are universal human experiences that can significantly impact on our mental, emotional, and physical well-being. Understanding the science behind them allows us to develop strategies to manage and even rewire our responses, leading to a healthier and more balanced life.

This chapter will explore:

- **The biology of worry and stress** – How our brain and body respond to stress.
- **The psychology of worry** – How our thoughts and beliefs influence stress levels.
- **The impact of chronic stress** – How long-term worry affects our health and relationships.
- **Practical management techniques** – How to break the cycle of chronic worry and stress.

The Biology of Worry and Stress: Understanding the Body's Response

When we encounter a stressful situation, our body activates the **fight-or-flight response**—an ancient survival mechanism designed to protect us from danger. This response triggers the release of hormones like **cortisol and adrenaline**, which:

✓ Increase heart rate and blood pressure to prepare for action.
✓ Heighten alertness to focus on the perceived threat.
✓ Suppress non-essential functions like digestion and immune response.

While this reaction is helpful in short-term, high-pressure situations (e.g., slamming the brakes to avoid a car accident), chronic activation of this response can be **damaging to both physical and mental health**.

The Impact of Chronic Stress on the Body

When worry and stress become a long-term pattern, the body **remains in a constant state of high alert**, leading to:

- **Increased risk of heart disease and high blood pressure**
- **Weakened the immune system, making you more prone to illness.**
- **Tension headaches, muscle pain, and chronic fatigue!**
- **Digestive issues, including ulcers and irritable bowel syndrome.**
- **Memory problems and difficulty concentrating**
- **Heightened anxiety and increased risk of depression**

This is why **learning to manage worry and stress isn't just about mental well-being—it's essential for long-term physical health.**

The Psychology of Worry: How Our Thoughts Shape Our Stress

Our perception of stress is just as important as the actual stressor itself. **Two people can experience the same situation but respond very differently based on their thoughts, beliefs, and mindset.**

Common Psychological Traps that Increase Stress

◆ **Catastrophizing** – Expecting the worst-case scenario to happen.
◆ **Overgeneralization** – Believing that one bad experience will lead to a pattern of failure.
◆ **Perfectionism** – Setting impossible standards and stressing over every mistake.

- **All-or-Nothing Thinking** – Seeing situations as either complete success or total failure, with no middle ground.
- **Rumination** – Replaying negative events over and over instead of letting them go.

When we get stuck in these thought patterns, we create **mental stress loops** that keep us in a cycle of worry. The key to breaking free is **learning to challenge and reframe negative thoughts**.

How Worry and Stress Affect Daily Life

Chronic worry doesn't just impact our body and mind—it can influence **every aspect of life**:

- **Relationships:** Stress can make us irritable, emotionally distant, or overly dependent on others for reassurance.
- **Career and Productivity:** Excessive worry can lead to procrastination, burnout, and difficulty focusing.
- **Decision-Making:** Fear-driven thinking makes it harder to make clear, rational choices.
- **Self-Confidence:** Constant worry can lead to self-doubt and feelings of inadequacy.

Recognizing these patterns allows us to **interrupt the cycle and replace stress with healthier coping mechanisms**.

Breaking the Cycle: Strategies for Managing Worry and Stress

The good news? **We can train our brains and bodies to respond differently to stress.** Here are **science-backed techniques** to reduce chronic worry:

1. Reframe Your Thoughts

Instead of "What if I fail?" try asking, **"What if I succeed?"** Challenging negative thoughts helps shift your mindset.

2. Practice Mindfulness and Deep Breathing

Mindfulness trains your brain to stay in the present moment rather than obsessing over past or future worries. Try deep breathing exercises to calm the nervous system.

3. Get Physically Active

Exercise releases **endorphins**, which act as natural stress relievers. Even a short walk can help lower cortisol levels.

4. Create a Problem-Solving Plan

Instead of **dwelling on worries**, focus on what's within your control. Write down the problem and list possible solutions.

5. Set Boundaries with Stressful Triggers

Identify what increases your stress (e.g., toxic relationships, social media, overworking) and set limits to protect your mental health.

6. Engage in Relaxation Techniques

Try **progressive muscle relaxation, guided meditation, or journaling** to help release built-up tension.

7. Improve Sleep Habits

Lack of sleep makes stress worse. Establish a nighttime routine that promotes relaxation.

8. Seek Support When Needed

Talking to a **trusted friend, mentor, or counselor** can provide perspective and emotional relief.

9. Reduce Stimulants Like Caffeine and Alcohol

Both can increase anxiety levels. Try herbal teas, water, or natural stress-reducing supplements like magnesium.

10. Focus on Gratitude and Positivity

Listing **3 things you're grateful for daily** can shift focus from worry to appreciation, helping retrain the brain for positivity.

10-Step Daily Practice Plan for Managing Worry & Stress

To put these strategies into action, here's a simple **daily routine** to help break the cycle of worry:

✅ **Morning:**

1. Start the day with a **5-minute-deep breathing or mindfulness exercise**.
2. Set **3 daily priorities** to create focus.
3. Reframe any worries using **positive self-talk**.

✅ **Midday:**

4. Take a **10-minute walk or stretch break** to reduce stress buildup.
5. Check-in with yourself: Are you caught in negative thinking? Adjust as needed.
6. Hydrate and nourish your body to maintain energy.

✅ **Evening:**

7. Practice **gratitude journaling**—write 3 things you're grateful for.
8. Limit screen time before bed to avoid mental overstimulation.
9. Do a **body scan relaxation exercise** to release tension.
10. Set a positive intention for tomorrow.

Final Thoughts: Taking Control of Worry and Stress

Worry and stress are natural human experiences, but they don't have to control your life. By understanding the **science behind stress**, recognizing **destructive thought patterns**, and implementing **healthy coping strategies**, you can begin to rewire your brain for peace and resilience.

Start small—pick one or two techniques from this chapter and integrate them into your daily life. Over time, these small changes will add up, leading to **a stronger, calmer, and more focused mindset**.

Next Steps: Reflection & Action

1. **Identify Your Triggers** – What situations cause you the most worry and stress?
2. **Practice One Stress-Relief Technique Daily** – Which strategy can you start using today?
3. **Challenge a Negative Thought** – Rewrite a recent worry using a more positive or neutral perspective.

Example: Rickey's Journey with CBT

Background:
Rickey is a 35-year-old man with no kids who has been struggling with excessive worry about his job security and financial stability. He constantly fears losing his job and wonders how he will support his wife if that happens. His mind often spirals into worst-case scenarios—what if he can't find another job? What if his wife leaves him because of financial struggles? These thoughts have been keeping him up at night, leading to fatigue, stress, and difficulty concentrating at work.

Step 1: Identifying Negative Thought Patterns
In his CBT sessions, Rickey learns to **identify** his automatic negative thoughts. His therapist helps him recognize patterns like:

- **Catastrophizing** – Assuming the worst will happen (e.g., "If I lose my job, I'll never find another one, and my wife will leave me.")
- **All-or-Nothing Thinking** – Viewing things in extremes (e.g., "Either I'm financially stable, or I'm a failure.")
- **Mind-Reading** – Believing he knows what others are thinking (e.g., "My wife probably thinks I'm not good enough.")

Step 2: Challenging & Reframing Thoughts
Rickey's therapist teaches him how to challenge these thoughts by asking:

- **Is this thought realistic?** "Have I lost my job? No. Am I actually on the verge of being fired? No."
- **What's the evidence?** "I have a solid work record, no recent warnings, and my boss hasn't given any indication of job loss."
- **What's a more balanced perspective?** "Even if I did lose my job, I have skills and experience to find another one. My wife loves me for more than just financial reasons."

Step 3: Developing Coping Strategies
To help manage his worry, Rickey practices:

- **Mindfulness & Relaxation** – Using deep breathing and guided meditation to stay present.
- **Problem-Solving Techniques** – Creating a financial backup plan, updating his resume, and networking to ease his job concerns.
- **Behavioral Activation** – Engaging in hobbies and social activities to prevent excessive worry.

Step 4: Practicing Exposure Therapy
Instead of avoiding thoughts about job loss, Rickey practices **gradual exposure** by writing down his fears and rational responses. Over time, this helps him desensitize worry triggers.

Outcome:
After several weeks, Rickey notices that his worries **don't consume him** as much. He's sleeping better, feeling more in control, and realizing that his self-worth isn't just tied to his job or financial status. His relationship with his wife improves as he communicates more openly about his fears without assuming the worst.

CHAPTER 3: MINDFULNESS VS. WORRY

Mindfulness and worry are two distinct mental states that significantly impact our well-being. Think of mindfulness as a lighthouse on a dark and stormy night—it illuminates the present moment and guides us to clarity and peace. In contrast, worry is like a ship tossed about on turbulent seas, constantly battered by the winds of fear and doubt. While mindfulness helps us navigate the present calmly, worry drags us into the uncertainty of the future and the weight of the past, leaving us feeling adrift and unmoored.

Understanding Worry and Its Effects

Worry is a form of negative rumination, an excessive preoccupation with potential problems or concerns. It is a natural human response to stress, uncertainty, or past experiences. When we worry, our brains enter a state of heightened arousal, triggering the release of stress hormones such as cortisol and adrenaline. These hormones prepare the body for perceived threats, causing physical reactions such as:

- Increased heart rate
- Muscle tension
- Gastrointestinal distress
- Sleep disturbances

While short-term worry can be useful in motivating us to act, chronic worry can have detrimental effects on both mental and physical health. Prolonged exposure to stress hormones can lead to:

- High blood pressure
- Weakened immune system.
- Increased risk of heart disease
- Anxiety and depression
- Cognitive difficulties, such as trouble focusing and decision-making.

Additionally, chronic worry often results in maladaptive coping mechanisms such as avoidance, procrastination, substance use, and withdrawal from social interactions. These behaviors can create a vicious cycle, reinforcing worry and preventing effective problem-solving.

The Power of Mindfulness

Mindfulness is the practice of intentionally focusing on the present moment without judgment. It allows us to observe our thoughts and emotions without becoming overwhelmed by them. Mindfulness can be cultivated through various techniques, including:

- Meditation
- Pilates
- Deep breathing exercises
- Tai chi
- Guided visualization

Unlike worry, which keeps us trapped in hypothetical scenarios, mindfulness anchors us in the present, reducing stress and promoting emotional balance. Scientific studies have shown that mindfulness positively affects both the mind and body. Some key benefits include:

Physical Benefits:

- Lowers blood pressure.
- Strengthens the immune system.
- Reduces chronic pain.
- Improves sleep quality.

Cognitive Benefits:

- Increase focus and concentration.
- Enhance decision-making skills.
- Strengthens emotional regulation.
- Promotes neuroplasticity, increasing gray matter in the brain.

Emotional and Spiritual Benefits:

- Enhance self-awareness!
- Fosters a sense of inner peace and connection.
- Improve coping with mechanisms for difficult situations!
- Cultivates gratitude and resilience.

Bridging the Gap: Moving from Worry to Mindfulness

Transitioning from a habit of chronic worry to a state of mindfulness requires intentional practice and patience. Below are practical steps to help shift from worry to mindfulness:

1. **Awareness of Worry Patterns:** Acknowledge when you are worrying excessively and identify the triggers.
2. **Practice Deep Breathing:** Engage in deep breathing exercises to calm the nervous system.
3. **Use Grounding Techniques:** Focus on your five senses to bring your awareness back to the present moment.
4. **Engage in Mindful Activities:** Incorporate activities such as mindful walking, journaling, or creative expression.
5. **Develop a Gratitude Practice:** Shift focuses from worries to appreciation for the present moment.
6. **Challenge Negative Thoughts:** Reframe anxious thoughts by questioning their validity.
7. **Establish a Mindfulness Routine:** Set aside time each day for meditation or relaxation exercises.
8. **Reduce Stimulants and Stressors:** Limit caffeine intake and create a calming environment.
9. **Seeking Support:** Talk to a trusted friend, mentor, or professional to gain perspective.
10. **Prioritize Self-Care:** Ensure a balanced lifestyle with proper nutrition, exercise, and restful sleep.

Conclusion

Mindfulness and worry represent two opposing mental habits—one fosters peace and resilience, while the other fuels anxiety and stress. By actively choosing mindfulness over worry, individuals can enhance their mental clarity, emotional stability, and overall well-being. Although eliminating worry completely may not be possible, learning to manage it through mindfulness can lead to a more fulfilling and serene life.

Chart comparing words related to *Mindfulness* **and** *Worry*:

Mindfulness	Worry
Present	Future-focused
Acceptance	Resistance
Peace	Anxiety
Awareness	Overthinking
Clarity	Doubt
Gratitude	Regret
Patience	Impatience
Focus	Distraction
Calm	Tension
Trust	Fear

Now, here's a side-by-side comparison of *Mindful Affirmations* vs. *Worrisome Thoughts*:

Mindfulness (Affirmations)	Worry (Anxious Thoughts)
"I am present at this moment."	"What if something bad happens tomorrow?"
"I trust that things will work out."	"I'm not sure I can handle this."
"I release what I cannot control."	"I have to figure out everything right now."
"I am doing my best, and that is enough."	"I'll never be good enough."
"I breathe in calm and exhale stress."	"I feel like everything is falling apart."
"I focus on what I can change."	"I wish I had done things differently."
"I accept myself as I am. As I grow"	"People probably think I'm failing."
"I choose to respond, not react."	"I don't know how to deal with this."
"I am safe at this moment."	"What if something goes wrong?"
"I embrace uncertainty with confidence."	"I can't stop thinking about worst-case scenarios."

Ricky's Crossroads Example: Worry vs. Mindfulness

Ricky sometimes feels insecure and less than a man because he cannot fully provide for his oldest son. There have been times when people called him a bum, saying he's not a good father because he struggles financially. Ricky has always been in his son's life since birth, but co-parenting has not been easy. He's had different jobs, yet stability seems just out of reach. No matter how much he holds himself accountable, it feels like he's always battling to stay afloat, just so he can support his son and be present in his life.

The Path of Worry

Ricky can allow worry to consume him. He can dwell on what people say—how they judge him for being behind on child support, how they label him as inadequate. He can fixate on his insecurities as a man, questioning his worth as a father. He can spiral into thoughts about his son's mother being in another relationship, wondering if his son will see the other man as more of a father figure. He can sit in sadness, fearing that his son will perceive him differently based on what others say.

If Ricky stays on this path of worry, it will only drain his energy. He'll be paralyzed by fear, self-doubt, and frustration, which will prevent him from taking meaningful action to improve his situation.

The Path of Mindfulness

Alternatively, Ricky can choose mindfulness. Instead of focusing on what others say, he can remind himself: *My financial situation will change. I am working toward a better future.* If he loses a job, instead of feeling defeated, he can analyze: *Why did I lose this job? Was it something I could control? How can I improve my stability?* This approach helps him find solutions instead of sinking into despair.

Through mindfulness, Ricky can focus on what he *can* control. If he feels he isn't spending enough time with his son, he can explore legal options for visitation. If he wants to build a stronger bond, he can find creative ways to connect, even if financial struggles limit his ability to provide materially. He can shift his mindset from *I'm failing* to *I'm growing*, turning every obstacle into an opportunity.

By choosing mindfulness over worry, Ricky can move forward with clarity and purpose. Instead of being trapped in fear, he can take action to create a better future for himself and his son.

CHAPTER 4: MINDFUL SELF-COMPASSION

Self-compassion is the practice of treating oneself with the same kindness, care, and understanding that one would offer to a good friend. It involves recognizing personal struggles, acknowledging imperfections, and responding to them with warmth rather than harsh self-judgment. Mindful self-compassion combines two essential elements: self-compassion and mindfulness. Mindfulness allows us to be aware of our thoughts and feelings in the present moment without criticism, while self-compassion encourages us to approach those experiences with gentleness and acceptance.

The Science and Benefits of Mindful Self-Compassion

Research has shown that cultivating mindful self-compassion can lead to numerous psychological and emotional benefits, including:

- **Increased Emotional Well-Being:** Practicing self-compassion enhances emotional resilience, helping individuals navigate life's challenges with greater ease and self-acceptance.
- **Reduced Anxiety and Depression:** Studies indicate that self-compassionate individuals experience lower levels of stress, anxiety, and depression as they approach setbacks with understanding rather than self-criticism.
- **Improved Relationships:** When individuals are kinder to themselves, they often extend that same kindness to others, fostering healthier relationships.
- **Greater Resilience in Difficult Situations:** By responding to failure and hardship with compassion, people can recover more effectively and maintain a balanced perspective.

How to Practice Mindful Self-Compassion

1. Cultivate Self-Kindness

Instead of engaging in harsh self-criticism, practice self-kindness. When facing difficulties, replace negative self-talk with gentle encouragement, just as you would for a loved one. For example, instead of saying, *"I always mess things up,"* try, *"I'm doing my best, and that's enough."*

2. Acknowledge Common Humanity

Remind yourself that imperfection is part of human experience. Everyone makes mistakes, experiences failure, and faces hardships. Understanding this can help reduce feelings of isolation and self-blame.

3. Practice Mindful Awareness

Be present with your emotions without suppressing or exaggerating them. If you're feeling overwhelmed, take a deep breath and observe your thoughts as if you were an impartial observer. Accept your emotions without letting them define you.

4. Engage in Self-Compassion Exercises

Daily practices such as journaling, meditation, or repeating positive affirmations can reinforce self-compassion. Write yourself a supportive letter during difficult times or practice guided self-compassion meditation.

5. Develop a Self-Compassion Mantra

Create a phrase that resonates with you, such as *"I am worthy of love and kindness, even when I struggle."* Repeat it whenever self-doubt arises.

6. Reframe Negative Thoughts

Challenge self-critical thoughts by asking, *"Would I say this to a friend?"* If not, replace it with a more supportive statement.

7. Set Healthy Boundaries

Being self-compassionate includes prioritizing your well-being. Learn to say no when necessary and establish boundaries that support your emotional health.

8. Practice Gratitude

Shift your focus from what you lack to what you appreciate. Keeping a gratitude journal can help you develop a more positive outlook.

9. Accept and Learn from Mistakes

Rather than dwelling on failures, view them as opportunities for growth. Ask yourself, *"What can I learn from this experience?"* and move forward with greater wisdom.

10. Seek Support When Needed

Self-compassion also means recognizing when you need help and allowing yourself to receive it. Whether from friends, family, or a professional, seeking support is a sign of strength, not weakness.

Embracing Self-Compassion as a Lifestyle

Mindful self-compassion is not about achieving perfection or eliminating negative emotions. Instead, it is about shifting the way we respond to ourselves in moments of struggle. By practicing self-kindness, embracing our shared humanity, and cultivating mindfulness, we create a more fulfilling and resilient life.

Next time you face a setback, pause and ask yourself: *"How would I comfort a friend in this situation?"* Then, offer that same compassion to yourself. In doing so, you will nurture a more positive and understanding relationship with yourself, paving the way for greater peace and personal growth.

A Real-Life Story from the Author: A Journey of Mindful Self-Compassion

There was a time in my life when everything seemed to fall apart simultaneously. I had to undergo emergency surgery, which left me unable to walk without assistance. The simplest tasks became difficult, and I had to rely on a walker to get around at the age of 38. On top of that, I lost my job, leaving me without an income to support my household.

The weight of these setbacks crushed me. I was angry, frustrated, and scared. I criticized myself harshly for not having enough savings in my bank account to prepare for an emergency like this. I kept replaying past decisions in my mind, wishing I had done things differently. I felt like I had failed—not just myself, but my children and the people who depended on me. I told myself I should have been smarter, more prepared, and in a better position to handle life's unexpected blows.

The negative thoughts consumed me. I questioned my worth, my abilities, and my future. I worried that I would never regain my strength, and that I would never be able to provide the life I wanted for my children. It felt like I was trapped in a never-ending cycle of self-blame and regret.

But then, something shifted. I realized that if I continued down this path, it would only lead to deeper depression, more stress, and possibly even worse health issues. I had a choice: I could drown in self-criticism, or I could practice mindful self-compassion and take control of my mindset.

Instead of tearing myself down, I started asking, *what can I learn from this? How can I grow?* I began acknowledging my struggles without judgment. I reminded myself that I was human, that setbacks happen to everyone, and that I had the power to turn this obstacle into an opportunity. I told myself; *this situation does not define me. My response to it does.*

Rather than dwelling on my past financial mistakes, I shifted my focus to learning better money management skills. I began setting financial goals and creating a plan to build savings for the future. Instead of sinking into despair over my physical condition, I embraced my recovery as a journey—one that required patience, persistence, and self-kindness. I committed to every step of my healing, celebrating even the smallest progress I made each day.

Most importantly, I stopped speaking to myself with harshness and instead treated myself with the same compassion I would offer a friend in my situation. I reminded myself that strength isn't just about avoiding failure—it's about how we rise after we fall.

Looking back, I see now that this difficult period in my life taught me one of the greatest lessons: true resilience comes from self-compassion. By choosing to be kind to myself, to acknowledge my struggles without judgment, and to focus on solutions instead of setbacks, I transformed my mindset and my life.

To anyone facing their own struggles, I want you to know this: It's okay to feel discouraged. It's okay to be frustrated. But don't let those feelings consume you. Speak to yourself with kindness. Recognize your strength. And remember, every setback is an opportunity to grow stronger, wiser, and more resilient.

This is just one of my real-life stories. And if I can rise from my challenges, so can you.

10 Steps to Practicing Mindful Self-Compassion,

1. Acknowledge Your Struggles Without Judgment

Recognize the difficulties you're facing—whether it's health issues, financial struggles, or emotional hardships—without being overly critical of yourself. Accept that struggles are part of life and don't define your worth.

2. Shift from Self-Criticism to Self-Understanding

Instead of blaming yourself for setbacks (like not having emergency savings), use the experience as a lesson for future growth. Understand that mistakes are opportunities to learn, not reasons for self-hate.

3. Reframe Negative Thoughts with a Growth Mindset

When facing challenges (like your physical recovery), remind yourself that healing is a process. Instead of saying, *"I'm weak for needing a walker,"* say, *"I'm making progress every day, and I will regain my strength."*

4. Focus on Solutions, Not Setbacks

Rather than dwelling on problems, shifting your mindset toward solutions. If you lose a job, focus on creating a financial plan, learning new skills, or looking for new opportunities instead of feeling defeated.

5. Treat Yourself Like You Treat Others

You've always encouraged and uplifted others. Now, apply that same kindness to yourself. When you face hardships, speak to yourself with the same support and encouragement you would offer a close friend.

6. Develop Emotional Intelligence

Recognize and manage your emotions without letting them control your decisions. Instead of reacting with frustration or hopelessness, take a moment to process what you're feeling and respond with clarity.

7. Embrace Setbacks as Part of the Journey

Your past experiences (like surgery and job loss) could have led to deep despair, but you chose to see them as steppingstones. Every challenge is temporary—what matters is how you rise from it.

8. Use Mindfulness to Stay Present

Rather than worrying about the future or regretting the past, focusing on what you can control in the present moment. Practicing meditation, journaling, or deep breathing can help ground you.

9. Set Boundaries and Prioritize Your Well-Being

Understand that self-compassion also means protecting your peace. Set boundaries with toxic people, manage stress, and make decisions that prioritize your mental and emotional health.

10. Believe in Your Growth and Future Success

Affirm yourself that your circumstances don't define your mindset and actions do. Keep reminding yourself: *"I am resilient. I am evolving. My challenges are shaping me into a stronger, wiser person."*

CHAPTER 5: REFRAMING NEGATIVE THOUGHTS

Our thoughts shape our emotions, decisions, and overall well-being. When we engage in negative thinking, we reinforce patterns that can lead to stress, anxiety, and even depression. However, learning how to reframe negative thoughts allows us to shift our mindset, fostering resilience and emotional growth.

Reframing negative thoughts isn't about simply stopping them—it's about acknowledging them, evaluating their accuracy, and transforming them into constructive perspectives. By actively reshaping our thought processes, we can create healthier mental habits that support personal growth and emotional stability.

The Power of Thought Patterns

Our minds function like a feedback loop. When we habitually think negatively, we condition ourselves to expect negative outcomes. This mindset affects our actions, which in turn influence our reality. Over time, negative thinking can:

- Create a distorted perception of reality!
- Reduce self-confidence and motivation!
- Attract negative energy and experiences!
- Influence the development of negative character traits!

Conversely, developing the skill of reframing our thoughts can shift this cycle in a positive direction, allowing us to build resilience and strengthen emotional well-being.

How to Reframe Negative Thoughts

1. Challenge the Thought's Accuracy

Not all thoughts are facts. Sometimes, our emotions influence our perception, leading us to believe things that aren't true. To challenge negative thoughts, ask yourself:

- Is this thought based on facts or assumptions?
- What evidence supports or contradicts this thought?
- Would I say this to a close friend who is going through the same situation?

For example, instead of thinking, *"I'm a failure,"* evaluate the evidence. Have you utterly failed in every aspect, or are you experiencing a temporary setback? By questioning the validity of a negative thought, you can break the cycle of self-defeating beliefs.

2. Shift Your Perspective

Reframing a thought means looking at it from a different angle. Instead of saying, *"I'll never be good at this,"* shift the perspective to: *"I may not be good at this yet, but with practice, I will improve."*

This small change helps replace self-doubt with a growth-oriented mindset, fostering motivation instead of discouragement.

3. Focus on the Positive Aspects

Every situation, no matter how challenging, has elements that can be viewed positively. When facing a setback, ask:

- What can I learn from this?
- How has this experience made me stronger?
- What skills or knowledge did I gain?

For example, if you fail a test, instead of dwelling on failure, focus on what you did well and how you can improve next time. This mindset not only enhances problem-solving skills but also encourages continuous growth.

4. Practice Self-Compassion and Accountability

Self-awareness and accountability are crucial in reframing thoughts. Holding yourself accountable means recognizing when you fall into negative thinking patterns and taking steps to correct them. However, accountability should be balanced with self-compassion. Be kind to yourself as you work on changing these thought patterns.

The Impact of Reframing Negative Thoughts

When you master the skill of reframing negative thoughts, you cultivate a mindset that is solution-focused rather than problem-centered. This shift improves your:

- Emotional resilience
- Ability to handle stress.
- Relationships with others
- Confidence and self-worth

Reframing negative thoughts does not mean ignoring reality or pretending challenges don't exist. Instead, it allows you to approach life's difficulties with a mindset that promotes problem-solving, learning, and growth.

Takeaway

- **Reframing negative thoughts** means shifting your perspective to see situations in a more constructive way.
- **Challenge negative thoughts** by questioning their accuracy and considering alternative interpretations.
- **Focus on positive aspects** of situations instead of fixating on failures or obstacles.
- **Balance self-accountability with self-compassion** to foster personal growth.

By consistently practicing these techniques, you can transform your mindset, improve your mental and emotional well-being, and create a more fulfilling life.

Reframing Negative Thoughts: A Personal Story

There was a time in my life when I struggled deeply with codependency. I had developed strong feelings for a close friend, someone I cared about deeply. Although our relationship had always been platonic, I found myself wanting more. However, I wasn't in a position to be in a relationship—my finances were unstable, my life lacked direction, and there were many personal struggles I still needed to work through. But despite all of this, I found myself hoping for something that simply wasn't meant to be.

As time went on, I started to feel insecure. I wondered why she wasn't interested in me the way I was interested in her. When I realized she was drawn to someone else, my self-doubt deepened. I questioned my worth: *Am I not good enough? Why wouldn't she want to be with me?* These thoughts consumed me, filling my mind with negativity and self-criticism. Instead of appreciating the friendship we had, I allowed my thoughts to distort my reality, making me feel inadequate and unworthy.

But something shifted when I took a step back and started evaluating my perspective. I began to see my own value. I realized that not every connection is meant to evolve into something romantic. Sometimes, no matter how much we care for someone, they may not be meant for us in the way we imagined. This realization led me to understand that true friendship requires respect for boundaries. If I genuinely cared for her, I had to respect her choices and feelings. I also recognized that my emotional reaction wasn't just about her—it was about me. My codependency and unresolved abandonment issues were surfacing, and I was projecting them onto this situation.

Once I changed my perspective, I started taking positive action. I focused on working on myself, embracing the time I had to grow and improve in different areas of my life. Instead of seeing my single status as a flaw or something to be ashamed of, I reframed it as an opportunity. I took this period to reflect, heal, and strengthen my mindset, knowing that self-improvement would prepare me for the right relationship when the time was right.

The biggest lesson I learned from this experience was that rejection isn't always a bad thing—it can be a form of protection. It can guide us toward self-discovery, teaching us what we need to improve and what truly aligns with our purpose. Rejection forced me to look inward, to see my own worth outside of relationships, and to understand that not every connection is meant to be something more. Instead of allowing rejection to break me, I used it as motivation to build a stronger, wiser, and more self-aware version of myself.

Reframing my negative thoughts about this situation changed everything. What once felt like a painful setback became a steppingstone toward growth and self-respect. It taught me that our thoughts shape our reality, and by shifting our perspective, we can transform even the most difficult experiences into valuable lessons.

What Went Wrong (Challenges & Negative Thought Patterns)

- **Codependency Issues** – The attachment to a friend became unhealthy due to emotional dependence.
- **Unrealistic Expectations** – Falling in love with a friend without acknowledging personal readiness for a relationship.
- **Insecurity & Negative Thoughts** – Questioning self-worth based on someone else's feelings, leading to thoughts like *"Am I not good enough?"*
- **Ignoring Boundaries** – Struggling to accept that the friend was not interested romantically.
- **Abandonment Issues** – Projecting personal fears and past emotional wounds onto the situation.

What Was Improved (Lessons & Growth)

- **Shifted Perspective** – Realized that not all connections are meant to turn into relationships.
- **Respected Boundaries** – Acknowledged the friend's feelings and honored the friendship instead of pushing for more.
- **Increased Self-Worth** – Understood that rejection isn't a reflection of personal value.
- **Turned Rejection into Growth** – Used the experience as a lesson to improve emotionally, mentally, and financially.
- **Focused on Self-Development** – Prioritized personal growth in areas like emotional intelligence, finances, and self-awareness to prepare for a future healthy relationship.

5 Ways to Identify Codependency & Negative Thought Patterns in Relationships

1. **Overattachment to One Person for Emotional Validation**
   - You feel like your happiness and self-worth depend on their attention, approval, or presence.
   - You may feel anxious, upset, or even lost when they don't reciprocate feelings or attention.
2. **Ignoring or Disregarding Boundaries**
   - Struggling to accept their decisions or personal space, even if they've clearly communicated their feelings.
   - You may find yourself overanalyzing their actions, trying to convince them, or feeling rejected when they set boundaries.
3. **Experiencing Self-Doubt & Insecurity**
   - Constantly questioning yourself: *"Am I not good enough?" "Why don't they like me?"*
   - Comparing yourself to others and feeling unworthy when you don't receive the affection or attention you hoped for.
4. **Projecting Past Trauma or Fears into the Relationship**
   - Bringing in past abandonment issues, assuming rejection means you're unlovable or destined to be alone.
   - Reacting emotionally based on past experiences rather than the reality of the current situation.
5. **Neglecting Personal Growth & Self-Sufficiency**
   - Prioritizing the relationship or person over your own self-improvement, financial stability, or emotional well-being.
   - Feeling like you *need* them to feel whole rather than focusing on building yourself up independently.

5 Practical Ways to Overcome Codependency & Negative Thought Patterns

1. **Developing Self-Awareness & Acknowledge the Pattern**
    - Journaling your thoughts and emotions to identify when you're overly dependent on someone's validation.
    - Asking yourself, *"Am I seeking their approval to feel worthy?"* or *"Am I basing my happiness on their attention?"*
2. **Set & Respect Healthy Boundaries**
    - Recognizing when you're crossing emotional boundaries and learning to step back.
    - Practicing self-discipline by giving space when needed and respecting the other person's feelings without forcing an outcome.
3. **Shift Negative Thoughts to Self-Empowerment**
    - When rejection triggers self-doubt, replace thoughts like *"I'm not good enough"* with *"I am enough, and the right person will appreciate me."*
    - Reframing the situation as an opportunity for growth rather than a personal failure.
4. **Prioritize Self-Improvement & Independence**
    - Focusing on personal goals, career growth, financial stability, and emotional healing.
    - Engaging in hobbies, learning new skills, or surrounding yourself with supportive friends and mentors.
5. **Seeking Support & Professional Guidance When Needed**
    - Talking to a trusted friend, mentor, or counselor about your emotions and experiences.
    - Practicing mindfulness, meditation, or therapy to process past trauma and build emotional resilience.

CHAPTER 6: PRACTICAL STRATEGIES FOR MANAGING WORRY

Worry is a natural part of life, often triggered by everyday stressors such as work, finances, and relationships, as well as significant events like illness or loss. While occasional worry can be a helpful motivator, chronic worry can take a toll on our mental, emotional, and physical well-being. It can disrupt sleep, reduce focus, and drain our energy, making it difficult to enjoy life.

The good news is that worry can be managed effectively. By implementing practical strategies, we can regain control over our thoughts, reduce anxiety, and cultivate a sense of inner peace. This chapter explores research-backed techniques to help you navigate worry in a healthy and productive way.

1. Scheduled Worry Time

Rather than allowing worry to take over your entire day, set aside a specific time to address your concerns. Designate 15–20 minutes in the morning or evening to write down your worries and analyze them objectively. During this time, you can:

- **Identify the root cause** of your worries.
- **Brainstorm possible solutions** for issues within your control.
- **Acknowledge and release** concerns beyond your control.

This structured approach prevents worry from becoming a constant background noise in your mind. By externalizing your thoughts through journaling, you create space for clarity and problem-solving.

2. Practicing Mindfulness

Mindfulness is the practice of being present in the moment without judgment. Worry often stems from dwelling on past regrets or fearing the future. By grounding yourself in the present, you can break free from anxious thought patterns.

Mindfulness techniques include:

- **Meditation:** Focusing on your breath to calm the mind.
- **Yoga:** Combining movement and breathwork to relieve stress.
- **Body Scans:** Bringing awareness to physical sensations to stay anchored in the present.

Research shows that mindfulness not only reduces worry but also enhances emotional resilience, allowing you to respond to challenges with greater clarity and composure.

3. Cognitive Behavioral Techniques (CBT)

Cognitive Behavioral Therapy (CBT) is a proven approach for managing anxiety and worry. It focuses on identifying and reframing negative thought patterns that contribute to distress.

A key CBT technique is **cognitive restructuring**, which involves:

1. **Recognizing negative thoughts** (*"I can't handle this."*).
2. **Evaluating their accuracy** (*"Is there evidence that I can't handle it?"*).
3. **Reframing the thought** (*"I have handled challenges before; I can find a way through this too."*).

By consistently challenging unhelpful thoughts, you can rewire your brain to approach difficulties with a more balanced and rational mindset.

4. Physical Activity for Mental Clarity

Exercise is a powerful tool for managing worry. Physical activity releases endorphins—natural mood boosters that reduce stress and anxiety. It also provides an opportunity to clear your mind and redirect nervous energy.

Effective forms of exercise include:

- **Aerobic activities** like running, swimming, or cycling.
- **Strength training** to build physical and mental resilience.
- **Recreational activities** like dancing, hiking, or team sports.

Find an activity you enjoy and incorporate it into your routine to enhance both your mental and physical well-being.

5. Seeking Support and Professional Guidance

Managing worry is not something you have to do alone. Talking to a trusted friend, mentor, or professional can provide valuable perspective and guidance. If worry becomes overwhelming, seeking support from a counselor, social worker, or therapist can help you develop personalized coping strategies.

Professional guidance can:

- Offer **structured tools** to manage anxiety.
- Help address **underlying emotional triggers** of chronic worry.
- Provide **a safe space** to express concerns and fears.

Reaching out for support is a sign of strength, not weakness. No one has to navigate worry in isolation.

A Story of Transformation: Overcoming Worry

Rickey was a successful businessman, but despite his achievements, worry consumed him. He constantly stressed over work deadlines, finances, and even minor daily tasks. His worries affected his sleep, his relationships, and his ability to enjoy life.

Determined to break free from his anxious cycle, Rickey implemented practical strategies:

✅ He **set aside 20 minutes each morning** to write down his worries, allowing him to process them logically instead of letting them dominate his day.
✅ He **practiced mindfulness**, starting with five minutes of deep breathing each morning to center himself.
✅ He **sought cognitive behavioral therapy (CBT)**, learning to challenge negative thoughts and replace them with more constructive perspectives.
✅ He **committed to daily exercise**, finding that running helped clear his mind and relieve tension.

Over time, these small changes led to a significant transformation. By taking proactive steps, Rickey learned to manage his worries rather than letting them control him. His mindset shifted from one of anxiety to one of empowerment.

Final Thoughts

Managing worry is a process, not a one-time event. It requires patience, consistency, and self-compassion. While worry may never fully disappear, you can develop the tools to prevent it from controlling your life.

By implementing structured strategies—such as scheduling worry time, practicing mindfulness, using CBT techniques, staying physically active, and seeking support—you can regain control over your mind and emotions.

Each step you take toward managing worry is a step toward **unlocking serenity** in your life.

Takeaway: The MEELEVATE Approach to Managing Worry

To help you remember the core principles of managing worry, use the **MEELEVATE** framework:

♦ **M - Mindfulness:** Stay present and self-aware in your journey.
♦ **E - Endurance:** Build resilience to overcome obstacles.
♦ **E - Empowerment:** Take charge of your thoughts and emotions.
♦ **L - Learning:** Embrace a growth mindset for self-improvement.
♦ **E - Emotional Resilience:** Adapt and thrive despite challenges.
♦ **V - Vision:** Set clear goals to guide your path.
♦ **A - Authenticity:** Stay true to your values and beliefs.
♦ **T - Transformation:** Strive for continuous self-improvement.
♦ **E - Empathy:** Practice compassion for yourself and others.

By applying these strategies and principles, you can take meaningful steps toward managing worry and cultivating inner peace.

CHAPTER 7: THE ROLE OF EMOTIONS IN WORRY

Worry is a natural emotional response to uncertainty, potential threats, or unresolved problems. While some level of worry can be beneficial—motivating us to prepare for challenges or avoid risks—excessive worry can take a toll on our mental and physical well-being.

At the heart of worry lies emotion. Our feelings influence the way we perceive situations, react to uncertainty, and manage stress. Understanding the role emotions play in worry can empower us to regulate our responses, develop healthier coping mechanisms, and ultimately reduce the impact of excessive worry in our lives.

How Emotions Drive Worry

Emotions shape our perception of the world, guiding our thoughts and behaviors. When faced with uncertainty, emotions such as **fear, anxiety, and vulnerability** can amplify our tendency to worry. Conversely, emotions like **confidence, resilience, and self-trust** can help us manage worry more effectively.

◆ **Fear & Uncertainty → Increased Worry:** Fear of failure, rejection, or danger can cause our minds to fixate on worst-case scenarios, leading to excessive worry.

◆ **Confidence & Control → Reduced Worry:** When we feel capable and in control, we are more likely to address challenges proactively rather than dwell on potential problems.

Our emotional state also affects how we respond to worry. If we feel anxious or overwhelmed, we may engage in avoidance behaviors—procrastinating, shutting down, or distracting ourselves instead of addressing the root cause of our worry. On the other hand, when we feel calm and self-assured, we are more likely to approach our concerns with logic and problem-solving skills.

Strategies for Managing Emotions & Reducing Worry

Emotions are powerful, but they don't have to control us. By learning to identify, regulate, and process our emotions effectively, we can reduce excessive worry and cultivate emotional resilience.

1. Identifying & Labeling Emotions

A crucial step in managing worry is recognizing the specific emotions fueling it. Instead of simply saying, "I feel anxious," try breaking it down:

- **What specific emotions am I experiencing?** (Fear? Frustration? Guilt?)
- **What triggered these emotions?**
- **How do they influence my thoughts and behaviors?**

Research shows that labeling emotions helps reduce their intensity. Instead of letting worry spiral out of control, we can take a step back, observe our feelings, and gain clarity on how to respond effectively.

2. Practicing Mindfulness

Mindfulness helps us stay present in the moment rather than getting lost in hypothetical worries about the future. By practicing mindfulness, we can observe our emotions without becoming overwhelmed by them.

Simple mindfulness techniques include:
✅ **Deep Breathing:** Slowing down your breath to activate a sense of calm.
✅ **Grounding Exercises:** Using your senses to bring yourself back to the present.
✅ **Body Scans:** Paying attention to physical sensations to release tension.

By incorporating mindfulness into daily life, we can create space between our emotions and reactions, allowing us to manage worry more effectively.

3. Using Cognitive Behavioral Techniques (CBT)

Cognitive Behavioral Therapy (CBT) is an evidence-based approach that helps individuals reframe negative thoughts and develop healthier emotional responses. CBT techniques include:

- **Cognitive Restructuring:** Challenging irrational worries and replacing them with more balanced perspectives.
- **Behavioral Activation:** Engaging in activities that promote relaxation and positive emotions.
- **Exposure Therapy:** Gradually confronting fears rather than avoiding them.

These strategies help us shift our mindset from one of helplessness to one of empowerment, reducing the grip of excessive worry.

4. Regulating Emotional Responses

Emotional regulation involves developing healthy ways to process and respond to our emotions. Techniques include:

💡 **Journaling:** Writing about your worries and emotions to gain insight and clarity.
💡 **Physical Activity:** Exercise releases endorphins, reducing stress and promoting emotional balance.
💡 **Connecting with Others:** Talking to a trusted friend, mentor, or counselor can provide support and perspective.

By regulating emotions, we create a foundation for mental resilience, making it easier to manage worry constructively.

A Personal Story: Transforming Emotional Reactions into Strength

Rickey had always been a high achiever, but with success came constant worry. He worried about meeting deadlines, making the right decisions, and maintaining his personal relationships. His emotions—fear of failure, frustration, and self-doubt—often dictated his thoughts, leading him to overthink and feel stuck in a cycle of worry.

Determined to regain control, Rickey started implementing emotional management strategies:

✓ He **identified his emotions** rather than generalizing them as "stress." When he recognized that his worry stemmed from fear of disappointing others, he was able to address the root cause.
✓ He **practiced mindfulness**, setting aside time each morning to focus on his breath and ground himself in the present.
✓ He **used CBT techniques**, learning to challenge negative thoughts and replace them with realistic, empowering perspectives.
✓ He **engaged in physical activity**, finding that a morning workout helped him reset his emotional state and approach the day with a clear mind.

Over time, these practices transformed the way Rickey handled worry. Instead of letting his emotions control him, he learned to navigate them with awareness and resilience.

My Key Takeaways On: The MEELEVATE Approach to Managing Emotions & Worry

To help manage emotions effectively, use the **MEELEVATE** framework:

- ♦ **M - Mindfulness:** Stay present and self-aware in your emotional journey.
- ♦ **E - Emotional Regulation:** Learn to process and express emotions in healthy ways.
- ♦ **E - Empowerment:** Take charge of your emotional responses instead of reacting impulsively.
- ♦ **L - Learning:** Develop self-awareness to understand the connection between emotions and worry.
- ♦ **E - Emotional Resilience:** Strengthen your ability to adapt to stress and uncertainty.
- ♦ **V - Vision:** Maintain perspective and focus on long-term emotional growth.
- ♦ **A - Authenticity:** Accept and honor your emotions without suppressing them.
- ♦ **T - Transformation:** Use emotional intelligence to create positive change in your life.
- ♦ **E - Empathy:** Cultivate understanding and compassion for yourself and others.

By embracing emotional awareness and regulation, you can break free from the cycle of excessive worry and cultivate a sense of calm, confidence, and control.

Final Thoughts

Understanding and managing emotions is key to reducing worry. By developing emotional awareness, practicing mindfulness, using cognitive strategies, and seeking support when needed, we can transform the way we respond to stress and uncertainty.

Managing emotions is not about suppressing them—it's about recognizing their role in our lives and learning to navigate them with wisdom and self-compassion. With consistent practice, you can cultivate emotional resilience, reduce worry, and create a more balanced, fulfilling life.

CHAPTER 8: BUILDING RESILIENCE AGAINST WORRY

Worry is inevitable, but it doesn't have to control us. Some people seem to navigate life's challenges with a sense of calm and control, while others are consumed by stress and anxiety. What makes the difference? Resilience—the ability to adapt, recover, and grow through adversity. By building resilience, we strengthen our ability to manage worry and reduce its impact on our lives. This chapter explores practical strategies to cultivate resilience and shift from merely coping with worry to thriving despite it.

The Power of a Growth Mindset

Resilience starts with a mindset. A **growth mindset** is the belief that challenges are opportunities to learn rather than threats to our well-being. When we embrace this perspective, we stop seeing worry as an enemy and instead view it as a signal sign that we need to act, adjust, or grow.

Consider a moment in your life when worry consumed you. Did it stop you from moving forward, or did it push you to find solutions? Imagine an entrepreneur who fears failure—if they let worry dictate their actions, they might give up too soon. But if they view obstacles as learning experiences, they keep going, refine their approach, and eventually succeed. Adopting a growth mindset helps us **reframe setbacks as steppingstones**, giving us the resilience to keep going despite fear.

The Importance of a Strong Support Network

Resilience is not built on isolation. Having a **support system**—friends, family, mentors, or professionals—can make a significant difference in how we handle stress.

For example, when I faced one of the most challenging times in my life, it was my close circle of trusted people who provided the encouragement, advice, and perspective I needed. Sometimes, just talking about our worries **lifts the emotional burden**, and at other times, guidance from someone with experience can help us find solutions we wouldn't have considered on our own.

Building a support network doesn't mean having dozens of people to turn to; it means having **the right people** who uplift, guide, and challenge you to grow rather than add to your stress. If you don't already have this, start by seeking out those who share your values and encourage your growth.

Developing Healthy Coping Mechanisms

Worry often leads people to unhealthy coping mechanism procrastination, avoidance, or numbing behaviors like overeating, drinking, or excessive scrolling through social media. Instead, **healthy coping strategies** help us manage stress effectively while improving overall well-being.

Here are three **powerful** coping mechanisms for resilience:

1. **Mindfulness & Self-Awareness** – Practicing mindfulness through deep breathing, meditation, or simply focusing on the present moment helps break the cycle of overthinking. Instead of drowning in "what ifs," we train our minds to focus on "what is."
2. **Physical Activity** – Exercise isn't just about fitness; it's one of the most powerful stress relievers. A simple walk, stretching, or a workout releases endorphins that **counteract worry and anxiety**.
3. **Intentional Reflection & Problem-Solving** – Instead of letting worries spiral, take a structured approach: write down concerns, brainstorm solutions, and identify small actions you can take immediately.

Setting Realistic Goals & Priorities

Worry often arises when we feel overwhelmed by responsibilities. A key strategy for resilience is **clarity**—getting clear on what truly matters and what doesn't.

A simple exercise: Every morning, list three priorities for the day. When we focus on what we *can* control, we shift from a reactive state to a proactive one. This builds confidence and reduces unnecessary worry.

Additionally, setting **small, achievable goals** helps build momentum. A goal like "I will meditate for five minutes today" is far more effective than "I need to eliminate all stress." The former is actionable, while the latter is overwhelming.

The Foundation: Taking Care of Yourself

Resilience isn't just mentality's physical, too. Sleep, nutrition, and self-care **directly** affect how we handle worry. When our bodies are depleted, our minds struggle more.

- **Sleep:** Lack of rest amplifies anxiety. Prioritize quality sleep by setting a nighttime routine.
- **Nutrition:** Avoid excessive caffeine or sugar, which can heighten stress.
- **Self-Care:** Engage in activities that nourish you, whether reading, listening to music, or spending time in nature.

Taking care of yourself isn't a luxury—it's a **necessity** for resilience.

Final Thoughts: Embracing the Journey

Building resilience against worry is **a process, not an event**. It takes time, practice, and consistency. However, by adopting a growth mindset, surrounding yourself with supportive people, developing healthy coping mechanisms, setting priorities, and taking care of yourself, you'll find that worry loses its power over you.

Try This: Resilience Journal Exercise

Each night, write down **one** challenge you faced during the day and how you responded to it. Ask yourself:

- Did I react with worry or resilience?
- What did I learn from this situation?
- What could I do differently next time?

Over time, this simple exercise will help you recognize patterns and build a stronger, more resilient mindset.

You have the power to turn worry into wisdom, fear into fuel, and challenges into growth. **Resilience is within you—now it's time to strengthen it.**

10-Step Plan for Building Resilience Against Worry

1. **Develop a Growth Mindset**
   Believe in your ability to learn and grow through challenges. Instead of seeing worry as a threat, view it as an opportunity for growth and self-improvement.
2. **Build a Strong Support Network**
   Surround yourself with supportive friends, family, and professionals who provide emotional and practical support. Sharing your concerns can help you gain perspective and find solutions.
3. **Develop Healthy Coping Mechanisms**
   Engage in mindfulness, exercise, and relaxation techniques to manage stress effectively. Finding healthy outlets for stress reduces anxiety and builds emotional resilience.
4. **Set Realistic Goals and Priorities**
   Focus on what truly matters and set achievable goals. Avoid overcommitting yourself and learn to say no to unnecessary stressors.
5. **Take Care of Your Physical and Mental Health**
   Prioritize sleep, maintain a nutritious diet, and engage in regular physical activity. A healthy body supports a resilient mind.
6. **Manage Your Time Effectively**
   Establish routines, prioritize tasks, and set boundaries to prevent feeling overwhelmed. A structured approach helps maintain control over daily responsibilities.
7. **Engage in Self-Reflection**
   Take time to analyze your thoughts, emotions, and behaviors. Identifying the root causes of your worries can help you develop personalized strategies to manage them.

8. **Practice Gratitude**
   Shift your focus from worries to appreciation. Acknowledge the positive aspects of your life to reduce stress and improve emotional well-being.
9. **Challenge Negative Thoughts**
   Learn to recognize and reframe irrational or negative thinking patterns. Developing a more balanced and positive outlook enhances resilience.
10. **Seek Professional Help When Needed**
    If worry significantly impacts your daily life, consult a therapist or counselor. Professional guidance can provide tailored strategies for managing stress and anxiety.

Illustrative Story: Anthony's Journey to Resilience

Anthony, a young professional, struggled with excessive worry. His concerns about work deadlines, health, and relationships affected his overall well-being. Unsure of how to manage his anxiety, he decided to implement the 10-step plan to build resilience.

- **Growth Mindset:** Anthony embraced the idea that he could learn from his struggles. He saw worry as a challenge rather than an obstacle.
- **Support Network:** He reached out to close friends, family, and a mentor, seeking advice and reassurance.
- **Healthy Coping Mechanisms:** He practiced mindfulness meditation, exercised regularly, and adopted deep-breathing techniques to calm his mind.
- **Realistic Goals and Priorities:** By breaking down tasks into manageable steps, he avoided feeling overwhelmed.
- **Self-Care:** He focused on sleep hygiene, improved his diet, and stayed physically active.
- **Time Management:** He structured his day, set clear priorities, and reduced unnecessary commitments.

- **Self-Reflection:** Through journaling, he gained insights into the patterns behind his worries.
- **Gratitude Practice:** Each morning, he listed three things he was grateful for, shifting his focus to positivity.
- **Challenging Negative Thoughts:** He identified irrational worries and replaced them with constructive affirmations.
- **Professional Help:** When he still struggled, he sought therapy, learning cognitive-behavioral techniques to manage his thoughts effectively.

Through this journey, Anthony transformed his relationship with worry. He realized that resilience is an ongoing process, requiring commitment and adaptability. His ability to manage stress improved, leading to a more fulfilling and balanced life.

Final Thoughts Building resilience against worry is a lifelong process. Experiment with different strategies to find what works best for you. By incorporating these steps into your daily life, you can develop a strong foundation for emotional well-being and long-term success.

CHAPTER 9: CULTIVATING INNER PEACE AND SERENITY

Inner peace and serenity are essential for a fulfilling life. They allow us to navigate life's ups and downs with grace and ease, finding joy and contentment in the present moment. However, cultivating inner peace and serenity can be challenging. Life is often stressful and chaotic, making it difficult to quiet the mind and find stillness. Yet, with dedication and practice, anyone can cultivate inner peace and serenity.

The Power of Mindfulness and Meditation

One of the most effective ways to cultivate inner peace is through mindfulness and meditation. Mindfulness is the practice of being fully present in the moment without judgment. It allows us to step back from our thoughts and emotions, recognizing them as transient rather than permanent. This awareness helps us detach from stress and anxiety, fostering a sense of calm.

Meditation complements mindfulness by training the mind to focus and quiet the constant mental chatter. Techniques such as breath awareness, repeating a mantra, or visualizing a peaceful scene can help center the mind and promote relaxation. Even a few minutes of daily meditation can significantly improve emotional well-being and reduce stress.

Practicing Gratitude

Gratitude is another powerful tool for cultivating inner peace. Shifting focus from what we lack to what we appreciate transforms our perspective, fostering contentment and reducing negative emotions. Practicing gratitude can be as simple as keeping a daily gratitude journal, where you write down three things you are thankful for each day, or take a moment to reflect on the positives before going to bed.

Engaging in Calming Activities

Various activities can promote inner peace and serenity, including:

- **Reading, Tai Chi, and Qigong**: These physical practices balance the mind and body, reducing stress and increasing well-being.
- **Spending Time in Nature**: Walking in a park, sitting by a river, or simply observing the beauty of the outdoors can be incredibly grounding.
- **Journaling and Creative Expression**: Writing, painting, or playing music provides an emotional outlet and self-awareness.

Developing a Lifestyle of Inner Peace

Cultivating inner peace is not a one-time event but a lifelong journey. It requires letting go of old patterns of stress and worry, replacing them with intentional habits that promote calm and balance. The goal is not to eliminate all stress but to develop resilience and navigate life with greater ease.

A Step-by-Step example story Guide for Rico to Cultivate Inner Peace

Step 1: Establish a Daily Mindfulness Practice
Rico can set aside a few minutes each day to focus on his breath, observing it without attempting to change it. This practice can be done in the morning or before bed to develop a habit of presence.

Step 2: Incorporate Meditation into His Routine
Starting with 10-15 minutes of meditation daily, Rico can find a quiet place to sit and center his focus. Guided meditation apps or recordings can also be helpful.

Step 3: Practice Gratitude Regularly
Rico can keep a gratitude journal, writing down three things he appreciates each day. Reflecting on positive aspects of life helps shift focus away from negativity.

Step 4: Engage in Physical Practices
Yoga, tai chi, or qigong can help Rico balance his mind and body. He can find online classes or videos to guide him through these exercises.

Step 5: Participate in Other Peace-Promoting Activities
Journaling, painting, playing an instrument, or taking nature walks can help Rico find moments of peace throughout his day.

Step 6: Reflect and Adjust
Each week, Rico should assess his progress and adjust his routine. He should practice patience, letting go of negative thought patterns, and focus on the present.

Final Thoughts

Inner peace and serenity are not destinations but lifelong practices. Anyone can cultivate a greater sense of peace and fulfillment by integrating mindfulness, meditation, gratitude, physical movement, and self-reflection into daily life. This journey requires patience, but it becomes a transformative way of life with consistency.

By applying these practices, Rico—and anyone seeking inner peace—can navigate life's challenges with a calm and centered mindset, ultimately leading to a more serene and meaningful existence.

CHAPTER 10: MAINTAINING A WORRY-FREE MINDSET: A LIFETIME PRACTICE

Throughout this book, we have explored various techniques and practices designed to help cultivate a worry-free mindset. We have examined the impact of negative thoughts and emotions on our well-being and how mindfulness, meditation, and self-reflection can empower us to overcome them.

However, as we reach the conclusion of this journey, it is crucial to understand that maintaining a worry-free mindset is not a one-time achievement but a lifelong commitment. It requires ongoing dedication, consistency, and the willingness to actively manage our thoughts and emotions.

Daily Mindfulness Practices

One of the most effective ways to sustain a worry-free mindset is through daily mindfulness practices. Whether through meditation, journaling, deep breathing, or simply pausing to appreciate the present moment, incorporating mindfulness into our daily routine allows us to become more aware of our thoughts and emotions. This awareness enables us to respond to challenges with clarity and composure rather than being consumed by worry.

Letting Go of What You Cannot Control

A significant source of worry stems from focusing on things beyond our control—such as the actions of others, unforeseen circumstances, or global events. Learning to accept that some things are simply out of our hands can be liberating. By redirecting our energy toward areas where we can make a difference, we free ourselves from unnecessary stress and anxiety.

Accepting Human Experience

It is important to remember that we are all human, and experiencing negative thoughts and emotions is a natural part of life. The goal is not to eliminate worry entirely but to recognize and manage these feelings healthily. Rather than resisting or suppressing them, we should acknowledge them, learn from them, and then let them go.

The Power of Personal Growth

Maintaining a worry-free mindset also involves continuously striving for personal growth. By regularly evaluating distractions, eliminating unhealthy habits, and setting intentional goals, we create an environment that nurtures peace of mind. Worry thrives in stagnation, but when we challenge ourselves to grow, we replace fear with confidence and uncertainty with purpose.

Mastering Your Thoughts

Worry has power only when we allow it to take control of our thoughts. It generates emotions and creates false narratives that can trap us in a cycle of anxiety and fear. However, by actively working on self-awareness and implementing the strategies discussed in this book, we can break free from this cycle.

Acting

Knowledge alone is not enough; we must apply it. Developing a plan and implementing solutions to address life's obstacles is key to overcoming worry. The tools provided in this book serve as a foundation, but true transformation occurs when we put these insights into practice.

Conclusion

Maintaining a worry-free mindset is a lifelong journey, not a final destination. It requires ongoing effort, self-reflection, and resilience. By embracing mindfulness, letting go of what we cannot control, accepting our human nature, and committing to continuous personal growth, we can cultivate a life of peace, confidence, and fulfillment.

You have the power to shape your thoughts and emotions. The choice to live free from unnecessary worry is yours—embrace it, practice it, and watch your life transform.

20-Step Plan for Personal Development and Maintaining a Worry-Free Mindset

1. **Acknowledge the Importance of Mindset:** Recognize that maintaining a worry-free mindset is essential for overall well-being and personal growth.
2. **Set a Clear Goal:** Define a personal goal for achieving and sustaining a worry-free mindset tailored to your unique life circumstances.
3. **Incorporate Mindfulness Practices:** Engage in daily mindfulness techniques such as meditation, journaling, or deep breathing to stay present and focused.
4. **Identify Negative Thought Patterns:** Reflect on negative thoughts and emotions, recognizing the triggers that contribute to worry and anxiety.
5. **Release Control Over the Uncontrollable:** Accept that some things—such as others' actions or global events—are beyond your control, and practice letting them go.
6. **Prioritize Self-Care:** Maintain a healthy lifestyle through adequate sleep, regular exercise, and balanced nutrition to support mental well-being.
7. **Seek Support When Needed:** Reach out to trusted friends, family members, or professionals for guidance and encouragement.
8. **Practice Gratitude Daily:** Cultivate a habit of gratitude by focusing on positive aspects of life, even during challenging times.
9. **Establish Personal Boundaries:** Learn to say no to commitments or relationships that do not align with your values and well-being.
10. **Improve Communication Skills:** Engage in active listening and express your thoughts effectively to build stronger relationships and reduce misunderstandings.

11. **Embrace Forgiveness:** Let go of grudges and practice forgiving yourself and others to free yourself from resentment and emotional burdens.
12. **Use Positive Self-Talk:** Replace self-criticism with affirmations and constructive self-talk to boost confidence and resilience.
13. **Adopt a Growth Mindset:** View challenges as opportunities for learning and growth rather than obstacles to success.
14. **Stay Present in the Moment:** Engage fully in each experience instead of dwelling on the past or worrying about the future.
15. **Develop Healthy Stress Management Strategies:** Explore effective coping mechanisms such as relaxation techniques, hobbies, or exercise to handle stress constructively.
16. **Practice Kindness and Generosity:** Perform acts of kindness toward others, fostering a sense of connection and fulfillment.
17. **Let Go of Perfectionism:** Accept imperfections and recognize that growth comes from progress, not perfection.
18. **Stay Open-Minded:** Be receptive to new ideas and perspectives, allowing yourself to learn and evolve continuously.
19. **Regularly Assess Personal Growth:** Reflect on your progress, celebrate achievements, and adjust your personal development strategies as needed.
20. **Commit to Lifelong Learning:** Understand that personal growth is an ongoing journey—be patient with yourself and embrace continuous improvement.

By following these steps, you can cultivate a mindset that reduces worry, enhances resilience, and promotes a fulfilling and meaningful life. Adapt this plan to fit your personal needs, and remember that your development journey is unique to you.

20-Step Plan: Unlocking Serenity—A Guide to Letting Go of Worry

Awareness & Understanding

1. **Recognize the Cycle of Worry** – Identify how worry impacts your life, relationships, and overall well-being.
2. **Understand the Science of Worry** – Learn how worry and stress affect your brain, body, and emotions.
3. **Identify Triggers & Patterns** – Recognize when and why you worry, and track recurring thoughts.
4. **Differentiate Between Productive & Unproductive Worry** – Learn to separate concerns that lead to action from those that create anxiety.
5. **Develop Self-Compassion** – Replace self-judgment with kindness and patience for yourself.

Shifting Mindsets & Thought Patterns

6. **Reframe Negative Thoughts** – Challenge limiting beliefs and shift your perspective to gain clarity.
7. **Practice Mindfulness** – Develop awareness of your thoughts and emotions through meditation and breathing exercises.
8. **Build Emotional Resilience** – Strengthen your ability to cope with stress by developing a growth mindset.
9. **Cultivate Optimism** – Learn how to shift from worry-based thinking to a hopeful, solution-oriented mindset.
10. **Let Go of Perfectionism** – Release the need for control and embrace imperfection as part of growth.

Taking Action to Reduce Worry

11. **Use Practical Stress-Relief Techniques** – Explore journaling, relaxation methods, and grounding exercises.
12. **Set Boundaries & Protect Your Energy** – Establish limits in relationships and daily life to minimize stress.
13. **Prioritize Self-Care** – Create a self-care routine that nourishes your body, mind, and spirit.
14. **Develop Problem-Solving Skills** – Learn how to manage difficult situations with a proactive approach.
15. **Practice Gratitude** – Shift your focus to appreciation and positivity to counteract worry.

Letting Go & Moving Forward

16. **Release the Past & Embrace the Present** – Learn how to let go of regrets and stay focused on what you can control.
17. **Find Meaning & Purpose in Life** – Connect with your values and passions to create a fulfilling life.
18. **Practice Forgiveness** – Free yourself from resentment and emotional burdens by choosing forgiveness.
19. **Embrace Change & Uncertainty** – Develop trust in yourself and the process of life.
20. **Maintain a Worry-Free Mindset** – Continue practicing these techniques daily to sustain inner peace and serenity.

Effective Techniques for Managing and Reducing Worry

There are several ways to manage and reduce worry. Some of the most effective techniques include:

✅ **Mindfulness:** Practicing meditation and self-awareness to stay present and reduce overthinking.

✅ **Relaxation Techniques:** Engaging in deep breathing, progressive muscle relaxation, or yoga to ease tension.

✅ **Exercise:** Incorporating regular physical activity to release stress and improve overall mental and physical health.

✅ **Problem-Solving:** Shifting from passive worry to active problem-solving by identifying challenges and taking action.

✅ **Time Management:** Prioritizing tasks and managing responsibilities effectively to prevent feeling overwhelmed.

✅ **Support System:** Seeking comfort and perspective by talking to trusted friends, family, or professionals.

✅ **Challenging Negative Thoughts:** Identifying and reframing irrational fears to develop a more balanced mindset.

✅ **Limiting Caffeine & Alcohol:** Reducing consumption of stimulants that can heighten anxiety and disrupt relaxation.

The MEELEVATE Approach to Overcoming Worry

A structured framework for personal growth and emotional well-being:

♦ **M - Mindfulness:** Cultivating self-awareness and staying present.
♦ **E - Endurance:** Building resilience to persist through challenges.
♦ **E - Empowerment:** Gaining confidence to take control of life.
♦ **L - Learning:** Adopting a growth mindset to improve continuously.
♦ **E - Emotional Resilience:** Strengthening the ability to thrive despite hardships.
♦ **V - Vision:** Setting clear goals and purpose to guide your journey.
♦ **A - Authenticity:** Living true to your values and beliefs.
♦ **T - Transformation:** Creating meaningful change for personal growth.
♦ **E - Empathy:** Fostering understanding and compassion for yourself and others.

A Personal Note from the Author

Thank you for purchasing this book—or even if it was given to you as a gift, I deeply appreciate you taking the time to read it. I believe that evaluating where we are in life is essential because worry can consume us in so many ways. We worry about our finances, our relationships, our children, our safety, and even what others think or say about us. We worry about whether we're good enough, about our insecurities, our health, and our future. If we let it, worry can take control, leading to stress, anxiety, and even depression.

But there's a difference between mindfulness—observing what we're going through and taking action—and the constant cycle of worry that weighs us down. Life is challenging, and while we can't always control what happens, we can control how we respond. I know I'm not alone in this struggle, which is one of the reasons I wrote this book. Worry has run through my family for generations. Growing up in poverty and facing financial hardship, not having the stability of a two-parent household—I know firsthand how worry can shape a person's mindset.

It took me years, becoming a father and reaching my late 30s, to understand worry and the power of letting it go. But letting go doesn't mean ignoring challenges—it means evaluating them in a way that helps us grow and elevate ourselves to our highest potential. Some days will be harder than others, but this is practice. We must be intentional about maintaining balance—mentally, physically, and spiritually.

Another important lesson I've learned is that we never know who's watching us and draw inspiration from how we handle life's struggles. Whether it's our children, our family, or even a stranger, we may unknowingly be role models. That's why learning to manage worry isn't just for us—it can also positively impact those around us.

Worry can create insecurities, damage relationships, and hold us back from the life we deserve. That's why I'm so happy you're here with this book. My hope is that you take something valuable from these pages because you are amazing, and I know you can overcome any obstacle and turn it into an opportunity.

Meelevate is not just a word—it's a lifestyle. And from Meelevate Books, Mr. Coach Davis, and myself, Rickey Davis Jr., I dedicate this book to you.

I also want to express my deepest gratitude to God, the Creator of this earth and universe, the Most High. I may not have liked every situation or battle I've faced, but I know each one was a lesson that helped shape me.

And to my three boys—I love you all more than words can express. You have changed my life, and I appreciate you beyond measure. I know I still have room to grow as a father, but I am committed to becoming the best version of myself—mentally, physically, spiritually, and financially.

To all my readers, thank you. I appreciate you. Keep striving, keep elevating, and keep pushing forward.

With gratitude,
Rickey Davis Jr. MEELEVATE BOOKS

Disclaimer

This book is based on my personal life experiences and extensive research. I want to be clear—I am not a therapist, psychologist, or licensed professional yet, but one day I will be. However, I passionately believe that self-evaluation and personal growth are powerful tools, and if you take the time to reflect and apply the principles in this book, it has the potential to help you on your journey.

I'm not claiming that this book will change everyone's life, but I do believe it can serve as a guide to help those who are willing to put in the effort and act. The insights and lessons shared here come from my own experiences—things I have personally lived through or witnessed firsthand. In addition to my life experiences, I have conducted research and utilized AI as a tool to assist in structuring this book in a way that is clear, helpful, and impactful.

I also want to take a moment to encourage those who have ever doubted their ability to write a book—you *can* do it. It took me a long time to find the confidence to start, but I made it happen. Don't be afraid to use every tool available to you, including AI, to help with grammar, structure, and storytelling. The most important thing is to share your story, your knowledge, and your perspective.

Never let anyone discourage you or make you feel like your goals are out of reach. If writing a book is your dream, go for it. You are capable of achieving whatever you set your mind to.

Rickey Davis Jr. Mr. Coach Davis

MINDSET ASSESSMENT OVERVIEW

Welcome to the Mindset Assessment. This tool is designed to help you evaluate your current mindset and identify areas where you can focus on growth and improvement. The questions within this assessment aim to explore your thoughts, behaviors, and attitudes towards various aspects of your life, including goal setting, motivation, emotional control, and personal development.

Please take your time to answer each question honestly. This assessment is for your personal reflection and growth.

You can choose to circle your answers directly on this page or write them down on a separate piece of paper to preserve your book. The choice is entirely yours. Your responses will give you valuable insight into your current mindset and can guide you toward the next steps in your personal development journey.

Thank you for your participation, and we hope this helps you unlock your full potential!

Meelevate Mindset Assessment

By Mr. Coach Davis

Instructions:

This assessment will help you evaluate your current mindset and identify areas for growth. Answer each question honestly based on your typical thoughts and behaviors.

Section 1: Goal Setting & Motivation

1. How often do you set clear and specific goals for yourself?
    - Very Often
    - Often
    - Sometimes
    - Rarely
    - Never
2. How motivated do you feel to work towards your goals?
    - Very Motivated
    - Somewhat Motivated
    - Neutral
    - Not Very Motivated
    - Not Motivated at All
3. How confident are you in your ability to achieve your goals?
    - Very Confident
    - Somewhat Confident
    - Neutral
    - Not Very Confident
    - Not Confident at All

Section 2: Emotional Control & Self-Awareness

4. How often do you feel in control of your thoughts and emotions?
   - o Always
   - o Most of the Time
   - o Sometimes
   - o Rarely
   - o Never
5. How well do you manage stress and anxiety in your daily life?
   - o Very Well
   - o Well
   - o Neutral
   - o Poorly
   - o Very Poorly
6. How often do you reflect on your personal growth and self-improvement?
   - o Daily
   - o Weekly
   - o Occasionally
   - o Rarely
   - o Never

Section 3: Growth Mindset & Adaptability

7. How often do you challenge yourself to grow and improve?
   - o Very Often
   - o Often
   - o Sometimes
   - o Rarely
   - o Never

8. How do you handle setbacks or failures?
   - See them as learning opportunities and push forward!
   - Reflect on them and adjust!
   - Get discouraged but try again later!
   - Feel stuck and unsure how to proceed!
   - Give up or avoid challenges!
9. How open are you to new opportunities and experiences?
   - Very Open
   - Somewhat Open
   - Neutral
   - Not Very Open
   - Not Open at All

Section 4: Mindfulness & Gratitude

10. How often do you take time to focus on the present moment?
    - Very Often
    - Often
    - Sometimes
    - Rarely
    - Never
11. How often do you practice gratitude for what you have in your life?
    - Daily
    - Weekly
    - Occasionally
    - Rarely
    - Never
12. How frequently do you take time for self-care and personal well-being?
    - Daily
    - Weekly
    - Occasionally
    - Rarely
    - Never

Section 5: Relationships & Support System

13. How often do you surround yourself with positive and supportive people?
    - Very Often
    - Often
    - Sometimes
    - Rarely
    - Never
14. How comfortable are you with setting boundaries in your personal and professional relationships?
    - Very Comfortable
    - Somewhat Comfortable
    - Neutral
    - Uncomfortable
    - Very Uncomfortable
15. How often do you seek guidance or mentorship to help with your personal growth?
    - Very Often
    - Often
    - Sometimes
    - Rarely
    - Never
    - **Final Reflection:**

What is one area that would you like to improve in your mindset? *(Open-ended question)*

Evaluation:

- **High Score:** Strong growth mindset, self-awareness, and resilience. Continue strengthening your mindset and mentoring others.
- **Moderate Score:** Some positive habits, but room for improvement in key areas like emotional control or goal setting.
- **Low Score:** Struggles with mindset, motivation, or emotional control. Consider seeking mentorship, support, or mindset coaching.

MINDSET ASSESSMENT ACTIVITY:

Instructions:
Read through the following prompts and take time to reflect on each question. Use a separate piece of paper to write down your responses. There's no right or wrong answer, this is an opportunity to understand where you are in your mindset and identify areas of growth.

---

1. Understanding Your Mindset:

Current Mindset:

- What do you believe about your abilities right now? Are they fixed or do you feel they can grow with effort?

Reflection:

- How do you typically approach challenges? Do you see them as opportunities for growth or obstacles?

---

2. Limiting Beliefs Identification:

Current Limiting Beliefs:

- Write down any negative beliefs you hold about yourself (e.g., "I can't do this," "I'm not good enough").

Reflection:

- How have these limiting beliefs impacted your actions and decisions?

---

3. Growth Mindset Practice:

Growth Mindset Mantra:

- Create a mantra or statement that represents your belief in growth and potential. For example, "I am capable of learning new things and overcoming challenges."

Reflection:

- How can you remind yourself of this mantra during moments of doubt or struggle?

---

4. Identifying Your Strengths and Weaknesses:

Strengths:

- What are your top strengths that you can use to overcome obstacles or achieve your goals?

Weaknesses:

- What are areas where you can grow? How can you work to improve them?

5. Setting SMART Goals:

Goal 1:

- What is one goal you want to achieve in the next 3 months? Be sure to make it Specific, Measurable, Attainable, Relevant, and Time-bound (SMART).

Action Plan:

- What steps will you take to achieve this goal?

---

6. Overcoming Fear of Failure:

Fear:

- What is one fear that holds you back from taking action?

Reflection:

- How can you reframe this fear and take it as an opportunity for learning?

---

7. The Impact of Your Mindset on Your Actions:

Impact:

- How does your mindset affect your behavior in various aspects of your life (work, relationships, health)?

Reflection:

- What changes can you make to shift your mindset toward growth?

Bonus Activity: Visualization

Visualizing Success:

- Close your eyes and imagine yourself achieving a big goal. What does it feel like? What steps did you take to get there?

Reflection:

- Write down what you saw in your mind's eye and how you can use that visualization to fuel your progress.

Final Reflection:

Growth Mindset Commitment:

- What steps will you take this week to develop a growth mindset? Write down three actions you will take starting today.

Closing Thought: Remember, this is an ongoing journey. Keep revisiting these prompts, and track your progress. Mindset is something that can be developed, and by taking these small steps, you are on your way to unlocking your full potential!

PERSONAL ASSESSMENT: UNDERSTANDING YOUR RELATIONSHIP WITH WORRY

Instructions:
This assessment is designed to help you understand your current relationship with worry. Answer each prompt honestly, and be open to the insights that arise. The goal is not to judge yourself but to gain awareness and begin the process of letting go of worry in your life.

Take your time with each section, and don't rush. Use a separate sheet of paper to reflect and answer each question. By the end of this assessment, you'll have a better understanding of how worry is affecting you and specific steps you can take to move forward with greater peace.

---

1. Identifying Your Worries:

Current Worries:

- What are the main things you worry about on a daily or weekly basis? (Examples: finances, relationships, health, the future, work)

Reflection:

- How often do these worries occupy your mind? Are there particular situations or triggers that cause them to resurface?

---

2. Impact of Worry on Your Life:

Physical & Emotional Impact:

- When you worry, how does it affect your physical body? (e.g., tension, headaches, trouble sleeping)
- How does it affect your emotions? (e.g., anxiety, irritability, sadness)

Behavioral Impact:

- In what ways does your worry influence your actions? (e.g., procrastination, avoidance, overthinking)

---

3. Worry vs. Action:

Control:

- What aspects of your worries are within your control? (e.g., actions you can take, decisions you can make)
- What aspects are out of your control? (e.g., outcomes, other people's actions)

Reflection:

- How often do you focus on things you can't control? How can you shift your focus to what you *can* control?

---

4. Reevaluating the Source of Your Worries:

Patterns in Worry:

- Are there certain thought patterns that repeat when you worry? (e.g., "What if I fail?" "What if something bad happens?")

- Do these thoughts tend to magnify situations or create unnecessary fear?

Reflection:

- How can you challenge these thoughts by rethinking or reframing them in a more positive or realistic light?

---

5. Letting Go of Worry:

Mindset Shift:

- What do you believe about worrying? Do you see it as necessary for problem-solving, or as something that drains your energy and hinders your growth?
- How would your life change if you could reduce or eliminate your worries?

Reflection:

- What would it feel like to live without the weight of constant worry? Take a moment to imagine the freedom that comes with letting go.

---

6. Building Your Worry-Free Plan:

Action Steps:

- What are three specific actions you can take to reduce worry in your life starting today? (Examples: practicing mindfulness, seeking support, setting boundaries)

Reflection:

- How can you incorporate these actions into your daily routine? Set a time each day or week to practice letting go of worry.

---

7. Trusting the Process:

Releasing Control:

- In what areas of your life do you find it hardest to trust that everything will work out?
- What does trusting the process look like to you? What steps can you take to begin trusting more deeply in your journey?

---

8. Embracing Serenity:

Serenity Visualization:

- Close your eyes and imagine a peaceful, worry-free moment in your life. What does serenity look and feel like? Where are you? What are you doing? Who are you with?

Reflection:

- Write down how you felt during this visualization and consider how you can bring more moments of serenity into your everyday life.

Final Reflection:

Growth Commitment:

- What is one thing you are committed to doing differently from today onwards in order to reduce worry and live with more peace?

Closing Thought: By taking the time to complete this assessment, you've already taken the first step toward releasing worry and embracing a life of serenity. Continue to revisit this assessment whenever you feel your worries creeping back in. Remember, worry is a habit, and with consistent effort and awareness, you can rewrite that habit for peace and calm.

Bonus Section: Worry Log

For the next 7 days, keep a Worry Log where you note down:

1. **What You Worry About:** (Briefly write what you were worrying about each day.)
2. **Physical Sensations:** (How does it feel in your body? Stress, tension, restlessness?)
3. **Reframing Effort:** (How did you try to shift your mindset or take action to reduce worry? What worked, and what didn't?)

At the end of the 7 days, review your log and reflect on patterns. What did you learn about your worries, and how can you continue to let go?

A Final Note to the Reader:

Thank you for being here and for taking the time to read and engage with this book. Your commitment to overcoming worry and embracing the tools we've discussed shows your strength and determination.

As a gift to you, I've left some blank pages on the back of this book. Use them however you like—whether for free notes, journaling, or just allowing your thoughts to flow. These spaces are for you to reflect on your journey, track your progress, and write down whatever comes to mind as you continue to grow.

Remember, these activities are not just for personal use—they can also be shared in group settings, should you find yourself in a position to support others.

You are amazing, and no matter what obstacles you face, keep pushing forward. Worry can manifest in many ways, but if we start teaching ourselves—and especially our children—how to manage it from a young age, we are giving ourselves the best chance at success and peace in the future.

I hope this book has served you, and I hope the extra pages provide you with the freedom to explore your thoughts and feelings. It was created with a lot of time, effort, and dedication to help you through your journey. The work doesn't end here. Continue to use this book as a tool for self-growth, and let the journey of overcoming worry be one you take with confidence.

Stay positive. Keep overcoming. You've got this.

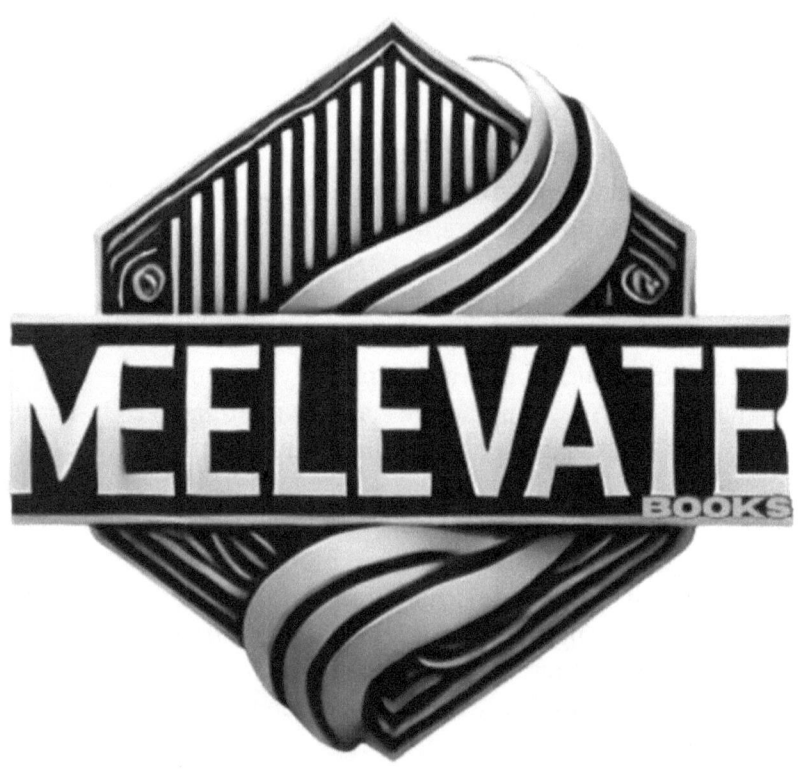

www.ingramcontent.com/pod-product-compliance
Lightning Source LLC
Chambersburg PA
CBHW031923240526
45464CB00022B/649